MENOPAUSE DIET COOKBOOK

Mary Dixon

TABLE OF CONTENT

CHAPTER ONE

Menopause Diet and Benefits

Following a menopause diet with benefits involves making dietary choices that can help alleviate menopausal symptoms and support overall health. Here's a guide on how to do it:

1. Consult a Healthcare Professional: Before making any significant dietary changes, consult with a healthcare professional or a registered dietitian who can provide personalized guidance based on your specific needs and medical history.

2. Balanced Nutrition:

- Lean Proteins: Include lean sources of protein like poultry, fish, tofu, legumes, and low-fat dairy in your diet. Protein can help maintain muscle mass and keep you feeling full.

- Healthy Fats: Opt for sources of healthy fats like avocados, nuts, seeds, and olive oil. These fats support heart health and hormone production.

- Fiber-Rich Foods: Incorporate plenty of fiber from whole grains, fruits, and vegetables. Fiber helps with digestion and can assist in managing weight.

- Calcium and Vitamin D: Maintain bone health by consuming foods rich in calcium (dairy products, leafy greens) and ensuring adequate vitamin D intake (sun exposure and supplements if necessary).

3. **Phytoestrogens:** Foods like soy products (tofu, edamame), flaxseeds, and whole grains contain phytoestrogens, which may help balance hormone levels during menopause.

4. **Hydration:** Drink plenty of water to stay hydrated, which can help with hot flashes and overall well-being.

5. **Limit Sugars and Processed Foods:** Reducing added sugars and processed foods can help with weight management and mood stability.

6. **Herbal Supplements:** Some women find relief from menopausal symptoms with herbal supplements like black cohosh, evening primrose oil, or red clover. However, consult with your healthcare provider before trying any supplements.

7. Portion Control and Mindful Eating: Pay attention to portion sizes and practice mindful eating to prevent overeating and maintain a healthy weight.

8. Regular Exercise: Combine your menopause diet with regular physical activity. Exercise can help manage weight, improve mood, and boost overall health.

9. Stress Management: High stress levels can exacerbate menopausal symptoms. Incorporate stress-reduction techniques like meditation, yoga, or deep breathing exercises into your daily routine.

10. Regular Check-ups: Continue with regular check-ups and screenings to monitor your health as you go through menopause.

11. Stay Informed: Keep up-to-date with the latest research on menopause and nutrition to make informed dietary choices.

12. Patience and Persistence: Understand that it may take some time to see the full benefits of dietary changes. Be patient with yourself and stay consistent with your menopause diet.

Remember that every woman's experience with menopause is unique, and what works for one person may not work the same way for another. The key is to tailor your diet to your individual needs and consult with a healthcare professional for guidance along the way.

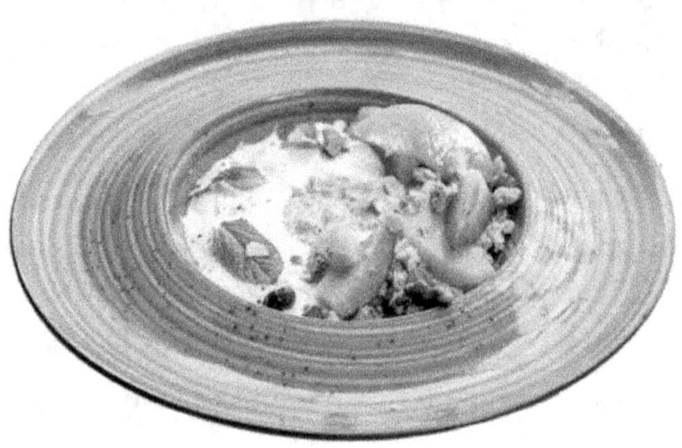

CHAPTER TWO

14-Day Menopause Diet Meal Plan

A 14-day menopause meal plan should focus on balanced nutrition, incorporating foods that can help alleviate menopausal symptoms and support overall health.

Keep in mind that this is a general plan, and it's essential to consult with a healthcare professional or a registered dietitian to tailor it to your specific needs and preferences.

Day 1:

- Breakfast: Greek yogurt with mixed berries and a sprinkle of flaxseeds.
- Lunch: Grilled chicken salad with mixed greens, cherry tomatoes, cucumbers, and a vinaigrette dressing.
- Snack: Carrot and cucumber sticks with hummus.
- Dinner: Baked salmon with steamed broccoli and quinoa.

Day 2:

- Breakfast: Oatmeal topped with sliced bananas and chopped walnuts.
- Lunch: Lentil soup and a side of mixed greens.
- Snack: A small handful of almonds.
- Dinner: Stir-fried tofu with broccoli, bell peppers, and brown rice

Day 3:

- Breakfast: Scrambled eggs with spinach and a whole-grain toast.
- Lunch: Quinoa and black bean salad with avocado and a lime-cilantro dressing.
- Snack: Greek yogurt with honey.
- Dinner: Grilled shrimp with roasted asparagus and sweet potato.

Day 4:

- Breakfast: Whole-grain cereal with almond milk and fresh strawberries.
- Lunch: Turkey and avocado wrap with whole-grain tortilla.
- Snack: Sliced apples with peanut butter.
- Dinner: Baked chicken breast with sautéed spinach and brown rice.

Day 5:

- Breakfast: Smoothie with kale, banana, chia seeds, and almond milk.
- Lunch: Quinoa and chickpea bowl with roasted vegetables and tahini sauce.
- Snack: Cottage cheese with pineapple chunks.
- Dinner: Broiled cod with a side of quinoa and steamed broccoli.

Day 6:

- Breakfast: Whole-grain pancakes with a dollop of Greek yogurt and mixed berries.
- Lunch: Spinach and feta stuffed chicken breast with a side salad.
- Snack: Cherry tomatoes with mozzarella cheese.
- Dinner: Beef and vegetable stir-fry with brown rice.

Day 7:

- Breakfast: Chia seed pudding with sliced peaches.
- Lunch: Lentil and vegetable curry with brown rice.
- Snack: Celery sticks with almond butter.
- Dinner: Baked trout with lemon, quinoa, and steamed asparagus.

Day 8:

- Breakfast: Scrambled eggs with diced tomatoes, onions, and bell peppers.
- Lunch: Grilled portobello mushrooms with quinoa and a side of mixed greens.
- Snack: Sliced cucumbers with tzatziki sauce.
- Dinner: Baked tilapia with a side of roasted Brussels sprouts and sweet potatoes.

Day 9:

Breakfast: Whole-grain waffles topped with Greek yogurt and a drizzle of honey.

Lunch: Spinach and walnut salad with grilled chicken and balsamic vinaigrette.

Snack: A handful of mixed nuts.

Dinner: Vegetable and chickpea curry with brown rice.

Day 10:

- Breakfast: Overnight oats with almond milk, chia seeds, and mixed berries.
- Lunch: Quinoa and kale salad with grilled shrimp and a lemon-tahini dressing.
- Snack: Sliced pear with cottage cheese.
- Dinner: Baked turkey meatballs with whole-grain spaghetti and marinara sauce.

Day 11:

- Breakfast: Smoothie with spinach, banana, almond butter, and almond milk.
- Lunch: Lentil and vegetable stir-fry with tofu and brown rice.
- Snack: Sliced bell peppers with guacamole.
- Dinner: Grilled swordfish with a side of sautéed spinach and quinoa.

Day 12:

- Breakfast: Whole-grain toast with mashed avocado and poached eggs.
- Lunch: Chickpea and kale soup with a side of mixed greens.
- Snack: A small bowl of mixed berries.
- Dinner: Baked chicken thighs with roasted asparagus and wild rice.

Day 13:

- Breakfast: Cottage cheese with sliced peaches and a sprinkle of sunflower seeds.
- Lunch: Quinoa and black bean stuffed peppers with a side of salsa.
- Snack: Sliced carrots with hummus.
- Dinner: Baked cod with a side of quinoa and steamed broccoli.

Day 14:

- Breakfast: Whole-grain muffin with almond butter and a sliced apple.
- Lunch: Lentil and vegetable curry with brown rice.
- Snack: Sliced cucumber with tzatziki sauce.
- Dinner: Grilled chicken breast with a side of sautéed spinach and sweet potato.

Remember to adapt the portion sizes and specific foods to your individual preferences and dietary requirements. Stay hydrated throughout the day by drinking plenty of water and herbal teas.

Continue consulting with your healthcare professional or dietitian to monitor your progress and make any necessary adjustments to your menopause diet plan. With time and consistency, you should experience the benefits of improved symptom management and overall well-being during menopause.

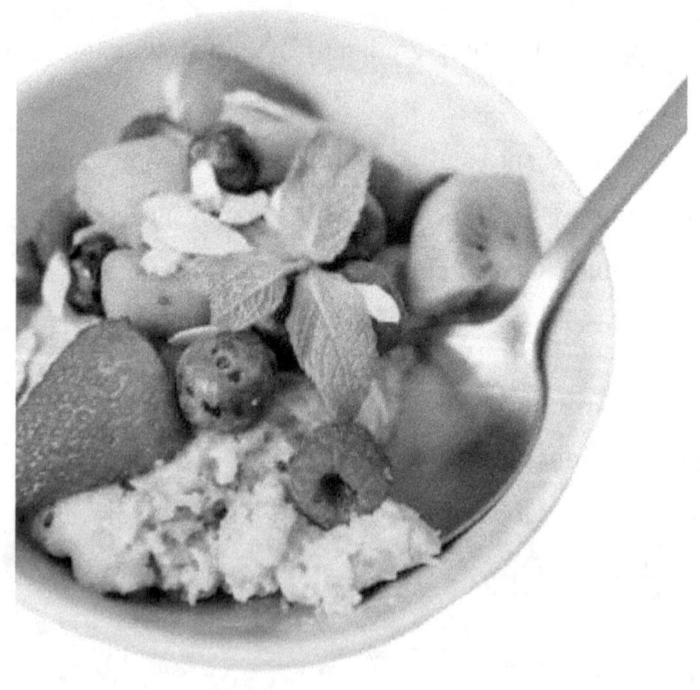

CHAPTER THREE

Menopause Diet Breakfast Recipes

1. Berry-Almond Overnight Oats

Overnight oats are a quick and nutritious breakfast option for busy mornings during menopause. The berries and almonds in this recipe provide antioxidants and healthy fats to support your health.

Ingredients:

- 1/2 cup rolled oats
- 1 cup almond milk
- 1/2 cup mixed berries (blueberries, strawberries, raspberries)
- 2 tablespoons sliced almonds
- 1 teaspoon honey (optional)

Instructions:

1. In a jar or container, combine oats and almond milk.

2. Add mixed berries and sliced almonds.

3. Stir well, cover, and refrigerate overnight.

4. In the morning, drizzle with honey if desired and enjoy.

Cooking Time: 5 minutes (prep time); overnight (chilling time).

2. Spinach and Feta Scrambled Eggs

Scrambled eggs with spinach and feta are a protein-packed breakfast that provides essential nutrients to help manage menopausal symptoms.

Ingredients:

- 2 large eggs
- 1 cup fresh spinach, chopped
- 2 tablespoons crumbled feta cheese
- Salt and pepper to taste
- Olive oil for cooking

Instructions:

1. Heat olive oil in a skillet over medium heat.

2. Add chopped spinach and sauté for 1-2 minutes until wilted.

3. In a bowl, beat the eggs, add salt and pepper, and pour them over the spinach.

4. Scramble the eggs and add feta cheese just before they're fully cooked.

5. Continue cooking until the eggs are set but still moist.

6. Serve hot.

Cooking Time: 10 minutes.

3. Greek Yogurt Parfait

Greek yogurt parfaits are a delicious and nutritious way to start your day. They're rich in probiotics and calcium, which can be beneficial during menopause.

Ingredients:

- 1 cup Greek yogurt
- 1/2 cup mixed berries (strawberries, blueberries, raspberries)
- 2 tablespoons honey
- 2 tablespoons granola

Instructions:

1. In a glass or bowl, layer Greek yogurt, mixed berries, and honey.

2. Top with granola for added crunch.

3. Repeat the layers if desired.

4. Serve chilled.

Cooking Time: 5 minutes.

4. Avocado Toast with Poached Egg

Avocado toast with a poached egg is a nutrient-dense breakfast that provides healthy fats, fiber, and protein.

Ingredients:

- 1 slice whole-grain bread
- 1/2 ripe avocado, mashed
- 1 poached egg
- Salt and pepper to taste

Instructions:

1. Toast the whole-grain bread.

2. Spread mashed avocado on the toast.

3. Top with a poached egg.

4. Season with salt and pepper.

5. Serve immediately.

Cooking Time: 15 minutes (including poaching the egg).

5. Chia Seed Pudding

Chia seed pudding is a no-cook breakfast option that's rich in fiber and omega-3 fatty acids, which can help with menopausal symptoms.

Ingredients:

- 2 tablespoons chia seeds
- 1 cup almond milk
- 1/2 teaspoon vanilla extract
- 1 tablespoon honey
- Sliced bananas and chopped walnuts for topping (optional)

Instructions:

1. In a jar, combine chia seeds, almond milk, vanilla extract, and honey.

2. Stir well and refrigerate for at least 3 hours or overnight.

3. Top with sliced bananas and chopped walnuts if desired.

4. Serve chilled.

Cooking Time: 5 minutes (prep time); 3 hours or overnight (chilling time).

6. Peanut Butter and Banana Smoothie

A peanut butter and banana smoothie is a quick and energy-boosting breakfast option, perfect for busy mornings.

Ingredients:

- 1 ripe banana
- 2 tablespoons peanut butter
- 1 cup almond milk
- 1/2 cup Greek yogurt
- 1 tablespoon honey (optional)
- Ice cubes

Instructions:

1. Add all the ingredients to a blender.

2. Blend until smooth and creamy.

3. Sweeten with honey if desired.

4. Serve immediately.

Cooking Time: 5 minutes.

7. Quinoa Breakfast Bowl

Quinoa is a protein-packed grain that can be used for a savory or sweet breakfast bowl, depending on your preference.

Ingredients:

- 1/2 cup cooked quinoa
- 1/4 cup Greek yogurt
- 1/4 cup mixed berries
- 1 tablespoon honey
- Chopped nuts (almonds, walnuts) for topping (optional)

Instructions:

1. In a bowl, layer cooked quinoa, Greek yogurt, and mixed berries.

2. Drizzle with honey.

3. Top with chopped nuts if desired.

4. Serve warm or cold.

Cooking Time: 15 minutes (including quinoa preparation).

8. Veggie Breakfast Burrito

A veggie breakfast burrito is a satisfying and savory option packed with vegetables and protein.

Ingredients:

- 2 eggs, scrambled
- 1 whole-grain tortilla
- 1/4 cup black beans, rinsed and drained
- 1/4 cup diced bell peppers
- 2 tablespoons diced onions
- Salsa for topping
- Avocado slices for garnish (optional)

Instructions:

1. In a skillet, sauté diced onions and bell peppers until soft.

2. Add scrambled eggs and black beans to the skillet and cook until eggs are set.

3. Warm the tortilla and place the egg mixture inside.

4. Top with salsa and avocado slices if desired.

5. Fold the tortilla into a burrito shape.

6. Serve hot.

Cooking Time: 15 minutes.

9. Tofu and Spinach Breakfast Wrap

Tofu and spinach breakfast wraps are a plant-based option filled with protein and nutrients to support your menopausal diet.

Ingredients:

- 1 whole-grain tortilla
- 1/2 cup firm tofu, crumbled
- 1 cup fresh spinach
- 1/4 cup diced tomatoes
- 1/4 teaspoon turmeric (for color)
- Salt and pepper to taste
- Salsa for topping (optional)

Instructions:

1. In a skillet, sauté crumbled tofu with turmeric, salt, and pepper until lightly browned.

2. Add fresh spinach and diced tomatoes to the skillet, cooking until spinach wilts.

3. Warm the whole-grain tortilla and place the tofu-spinach mixture inside.

4. Top with salsa if desired.

5. Fold into a wrap.

6. Serve warm.

Cooking Time: 15 minutes.

10. Blueberry and Almond Breakfast Quinoa

Blueberry and almond breakfast quinoa is a hearty and wholesome option that combines the goodness of whole grains, antioxidants, and healthy fats.

Ingredients:

- 1/2 cup cooked quinoa
- 1/4 cup blueberries
- 2 tablespoons slivered almonds
- 1 teaspoon honey
- 1/4 teaspoon cinnamon (optional)

Instructions:

1. In a bowl, combine cooked quinoa, blueberries, and slivered almonds.

2. Drizzle with honey and sprinkle with cinnamon if desired.

3. Serve warm.

Cooking Time: 15 minutes (including quinoa preparation).

Menopause Diet Lunch Recipes

1. Quinoa and Chickpea Salad

This quinoa and chickpea salad is packed with protein and fiber, making it an excellent choice for a nutritious and satisfying menopause-friendly lunch.

Ingredients:

- 1 cup cooked quinoa
- 1 cup canned chickpeas, rinsed and drained
- 1 cucumber, diced
- 1 red bell pepper, diced
- 1/4 cup chopped fresh parsley
- 2 tablespoons lemon juice

- 2 tablespoons olive oil

- Salt and pepper to taste

Instructions:

1. In a large bowl, combine quinoa, chickpeas, cucumber, red bell pepper, and chopped parsley.

2. In a separate small bowl, whisk together lemon juice, olive oil, salt, and pepper.

3. Pour the dressing over the salad and toss to combine.

4. Serve chilled.

Cooking Time: 20 minutes (including quinoa preparation).

2. Spinach and Feta Stuffed Chicken Breast

This stuffed chicken breast recipe is a protein-rich option with the goodness of spinach and feta, perfect for a filling menopause diet lunch.

Ingredients:

- 2 boneless, skinless chicken breasts

- 2 cups fresh spinach, chopped

- 1/4 cup crumbled feta cheese

- 1 clove garlic, minced

- Salt and pepper to taste

- Olive oil for cooking

Instructions:

1. Preheat the oven to 375°F (190°C).

2. In a skillet, heat olive oil over medium heat.

3. Add minced garlic and chopped spinach, sauté until wilted.

4. Slice a pocket into each chicken breast.

5. Stuff each breast with sautéed spinach and crumbled feta.

6. Season the chicken breasts with salt and pepper.

7. Heat more olive oil in the skillet, and sear each chicken breast for 2-3 minutes per side.

8. Transfer the chicken to a baking dish and bake for 15-20 minutes until cooked through.

9. Serve hot.

Cooking Time: 40 minutes.

3. Lentil and Vegetable Stir-Fry

A lentil and vegetable stir-fry is a plant-based lunch option rich in protein, fiber, and essential nutrients to support menopausal health.

Ingredients:

- 1 cup cooked green lentils
- 2 cups mixed vegetables (bell peppers, broccoli, carrots), sliced
- 2 cloves garlic, minced
- 2 tablespoons low-sodium soy sauce
- 1 tablespoon olive oil
- 1/4 teaspoon red pepper flakes (optional)

Instructions:

1. Heat olive oil in a skillet over medium-high heat.

2. Add minced garlic and stir for 30 seconds.

3. Add sliced vegetables and cook until tender-crisp.

4. Stir in cooked lentils, soy sauce, and red pepper flakes (if using).

5. Cook for an additional 2-3 minutes, ensuring everything is well combined.

6. Serve hot.

Cooking Time: 20 minutes (including lentil preparation).

4. Greek Salad with Grilled Shrimp

A Greek salad with grilled shrimp is a refreshing and protein-packed lunch option that includes plenty of fresh vegetables.

Ingredients:

- 1 cup mixed greens
- 8-10 grilled shrimp
- 1/2 cucumber, sliced
- 1/2 cup cherry tomatoes, halved
- 1/4 red onion, thinly sliced
- 1/4 cup crumbled feta cheese
- Kalamata olives (optional)
- Greek dressing (olive oil, lemon juice, oregano, salt, and pepper)

Instructions:

1. Arrange mixed greens on a plate.

2. Top with grilled shrimp, cucumber, cherry tomatoes, red onion, and feta cheese.

3. Add Kalamata olives if desired.

4. Drizzle with Greek dressing.

5. Serve chilled.

Cooking Time: 15 minutes (including shrimp grilling time).

5. Chickpea and Spinach Curry

This chickpea and spinach curry is a flavorful and vegetarian option packed with protein, fiber, and essential nutrients.

Ingredients:

- 1 can (15 oz) chickpeas, rinsed and drained
- 2 cups fresh spinach
- 1 onion, finely chopped
- 2 cloves garlic, minced
- 1-inch piece of ginger, minced
- 1 can (14 oz) diced tomatoes
- 2 teaspoons curry powder

- 1 teaspoon cumin

- 1 teaspoon coriander

- Salt and pepper to taste

- 2 tablespoons olive oil

- Fresh cilantro for garnish

Instructions:

1. Heat olive oil in a large skillet over medium heat.

2. Add chopped onion and sauté until translucent.

3. Stir in minced garlic and ginger and cook for another minute.

4. Add diced tomatoes, chickpeas, curry powder, cumin, coriander, salt, and pepper.

5. Simmer for 10-15 minutes, stirring occasionally.

6. Just before serving, add fresh spinach and cook until wilted.

7. Garnish with fresh cilantro.

8. Serve with rice or whole-grain bread.

Cooking Time: 30 minutes.

6. Salmon and Avocado Salad

A salmon and avocado salad is a delicious and omega-3-rich lunch option that supports heart and bone health during menopause.

Ingredients:

- 1 grilled or baked salmon fillet
- 1/2 avocado, sliced
- Mixed greens or spinach
- Cherry tomatoes, halved
- Red onion, thinly sliced
- Lemon-dill dressing (lemon juice, olive oil, fresh dill, salt, and pepper)

Instructions:

1. Arrange mixed greens on a plate.

2. Top with grilled or baked salmon, avocado slices, cherry tomatoes, and red onion.

3. Drizzle with lemon-dill dressing.

4. Serve chilled.

Cooking Time: 15 minutes (including salmon grilling/baking time).

7. Lentil Soup

A hearty lentil soup is a comforting and nutritious lunch option, providing plenty of fiber and plant-based protein.

Ingredients:

- 1 cup dried green or brown lentils, rinsed
- 1 onion, chopped
- 2 carrots, diced
- 2 celery stalks, diced
- 2 cloves garlic, minced
- 1 can (14 oz) diced tomatoes
- 6 cups vegetable broth
- 1 teaspoon cumin
- 1/2 teaspoon smoked paprika
- Salt and pepper to taste
- Olive oil for cooking

Instructions:

1. Heat olive oil in a large pot over medium heat.

2. Add chopped onion, carrots, and celery. Sauté until softened.

3. Stir in minced garlic, cumin, and smoked paprika. Cook for 1 minute.

4. Add rinsed lentils, diced tomatoes, and vegetable broth.

5. Bring to a boil, then reduce heat and simmer for 20-25 minutes, or until lentils are tender.

6. Season with salt and pepper.

7. Serve hot.

Cooking Time: 45 minutes (including prep and simmering time).

8. Turkey and Avocado Wrap

A turkey and avocado wrap is a quick and protein-rich lunch option that's perfect for when you're on the go.

Ingredients:

- 1 whole-grain tortilla
- 4-6 slices turkey breast
- 1/2 avocado, sliced
- Mixed greens or spinach
- Dijon mustard (optional)

Instructions:

1. Lay the whole-grain tortilla flat.

2. Arrange turkey slices, avocado slices, and mixed greens or spinach in the center.

3. Drizzle with Dijon mustard if desired.

4. Roll the tortilla into a wrap.

5. Slice in half and serve.

Cooking Time: 10 minutes.

9. Caprese Salad with Quinoa

A Caprese salad with quinoa is a twist on the classic with the added benefit of quinoa's protein and fiber content.

Ingredients:

- 1 cup cooked quinoa
- 1 cup cherry tomatoes, halved
- 1 cup fresh mozzarella cheese, diced
- Fresh basil leaves
- Balsamic glaze (optional)
- Olive oil, salt, and pepper for dressing

Instructions:

1. In a bowl, combine cooked quinoa, cherry tomatoes, and fresh mozzarella.

2. Drizzle with olive oil and season with salt and pepper.

3. Garnish with fresh basil leaves.

4. Drizzle with balsamic glaze if desired.

5. Serve chilled.

Cooking Time: 15 minutes (including quinoa preparation).

10. Tofu and Broccoli Stir-Fry

A tofu and broccoli stir-fry is a nutritious and plant-based lunch option rich in protein and fiber.

Ingredients:

- 1/2 block firm tofu, cubed
- 2 cups broccoli florets
- 1 red bell pepper, sliced
- 2 cloves garlic, minced
- 1/4 cup low-sodium soy sauce
- 1 tablespoon olive oil
- 1 tablespoon cornstarch (optional, for thickening)
- Cooked brown rice or quinoa for serving

Instructions:

1. Heat olive oil in a skillet over medium-high heat.

2. Add cubed tofu and cook until lightly browned.

3. Add minced garlic, broccoli, and red bell pepper. Stir-fry until vegetables are tender.

4. In a small bowl, whisk together soy sauce and cornstarch (if using).

5. Pour the sauce over the stir-fry and cook until it thickens.

6. Serve over cooked brown rice or quinoa.

Cooking Time: 25 minutes.

These 10 menopause diet lunch recipes offer a variety of flavors and ingredients that cater to your nutritional needs during this phase of life. Enjoy these meals as part of your balanced and supportive menopause diet.

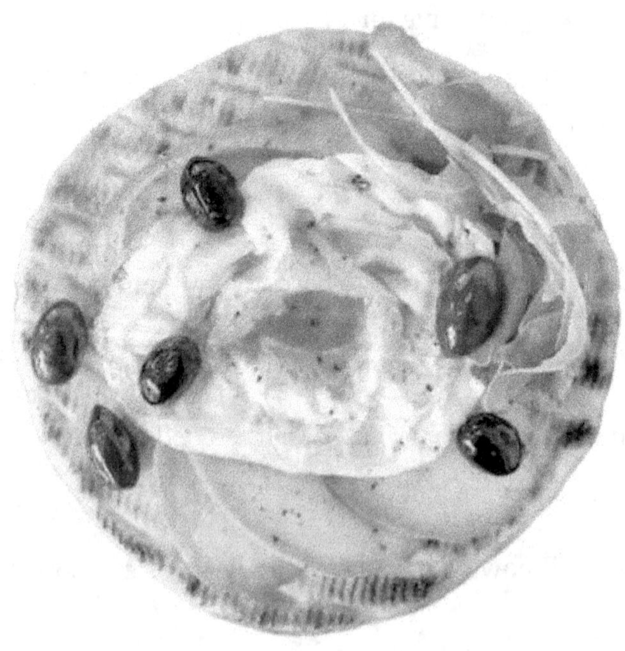

CHAPTER FOUR

Menopause Diet Dinner Recipes

1. Baked Salmon with Lemon-Dill Sauce

Baked salmon is rich in omega-3 fatty acids, which can help manage menopausal symptoms. This recipe is quick and delicious.

Ingredients:

- 4 salmon fillets
- 2 tablespoons olive oil
- 2 cloves garlic, minced
- Zest and juice of 1 lemon
- 2 tablespoons fresh dill, chopped
- Salt and pepper to taste

Instructions:

1. Preheat the oven to 375°F (190°C).

2. Place salmon fillets on a baking sheet.

3. In a bowl, mix olive oil, minced garlic, lemon zest, lemon juice, and chopped dill.

4. Brush the mixture over the salmon.

5. Season with salt and pepper.

6. Bake for 15-20 minutes, or until the salmon flakes easily.

7. Serve hot.

Cooking Time: 20 minutes.

2. Vegetable Stir-Fried Tofu

This vegetable stir-fry with tofu is a plant-based dinner option rich in protein and fiber to support a balanced menopause diet.

Ingredients:

- 1 block firm tofu, cubed
- 2 cups mixed vegetables (broccoli, bell peppers, snap peas, carrots)
- 2 cloves garlic, minced
- 2 tablespoons low-sodium soy sauce
- 1 tablespoon sesame oil
- 1 tablespoon cornstarch (optional, for thickening)
- Cooked brown rice or quinoa for serving

Instructions:

1. Heat sesame oil in a skillet or wok over medium-high heat.

2. Add cubed tofu and cook until golden brown.

3. Add minced garlic and mixed vegetables. Stir-fry until vegetables are tender-crisp.

4. In a small bowl, whisk together soy sauce and cornstarch (if using).

5. Pour the sauce over the stir-fry and cook until it thickens.

6. Serve over cooked brown rice or quinoa.

Cooking Time: 25 minutes.

3. Lemon-Herb Grilled Chicken

Grilled chicken with a lemon-herb marinade is a flavorful and protein-packed dinner option for your menopause diet.

Ingredients:

- 4 boneless, skinless chicken breasts
- Juice and zest of 2 lemons
- 2 cloves garlic, minced

- 2 tablespoons fresh herbs (rosemary, thyme, oregano), chopped
- Salt and pepper to taste
- Olive oil for grilling

Instructions:

1. In a bowl, mix lemon juice, lemon zest, minced garlic, chopped herbs, salt, and pepper.

2. Marinate chicken breasts in the mixture for at least 30 minutes.

3. Preheat the grill to medium-high heat.

4. Grill the chicken for about 6-7 minutes per side, or until cooked through.

5. Serve hot.

Cooking Time: 20 minutes (including marinating time).

4. Quinoa and Black Bean Stuffed Bell Peppers

Stuffed bell peppers with quinoa and black beans are a nutrient-dense dinner option packed with protein and fiber.

Ingredients:

- 4 bell peppers, any color
- 1 cup cooked quinoa
- 1 cup canned black beans, rinsed and drained
- 1 cup diced tomatoes
- 1/2 cup corn kernels (fresh or frozen)
- 1/2 cup diced red onion
- 1 teaspoon chili powder
- 1/2 teaspoon cumin
- Salt and pepper to taste
- Olive oil for drizzling

Instructions:

1. Preheat the oven to 375°F (190°C).

2. Cut the tops off the bell peppers and remove seeds.

3. In a bowl, mix cooked quinoa, black beans, diced tomatoes, corn, red onion, chili powder, cumin, salt, and pepper.

4. Stuff the bell peppers with the quinoa mixture.

5. Place the stuffed peppers in a baking dish, drizzle with olive oil, and cover with foil.

6. Bake for 30-35 minutes, or until the peppers are tender.

7. Serve hot.

Cooking Time: 45 minutes (including baking time).

5. Lentil and Vegetable Curry

A lentil and vegetable curry is a flavorful and plant-based dinner option rich in protein and fiber, perfect for your menopause diet.

Ingredients:

- 1 cup dried green or brown lentils, rinsed
- 2 cups mixed vegetables (bell peppers, broccoli, carrots), sliced
- 1 onion, finely chopped
- 2 cloves garlic, minced
- 1-inch piece of ginger, minced
- 1 can (14 oz) diced tomatoes
- 2 teaspoons curry powder
- 1 teaspoon cumin

- 1 teaspoon coriander
- Salt and pepper to taste
- Olive oil for cooking
- Fresh cilantro for garnish

Instructions:

1. Heat olive oil in a large skillet over medium heat.

2. Add chopped onion and sauté until translucent.

3. Stir in minced garlic and ginger and cook for another minute.

4. Add diced tomatoes, lentils, curry powder, cumin, coriander, salt, and pepper.

5. Simmer for 20-25 minutes, or until lentils are tender, stirring occasionally.

6. Just before serving, add mixed vegetables and cook until they are tender-crisp.

7. Garnish with fresh cilantro.

8. Serve with rice or whole-grain bread.

Cooking Time: 45 minutes.

6. Spaghetti Squash with Tomato Basil Sauce

Spaghetti squash is a low-carb alternative to pasta, and when paired with a fresh tomato basil sauce, it makes a light and satisfying dinner.

Ingredients:

- 1 medium spaghetti squash
- 2 cups diced tomatoes (canned or fresh)
- 1/4 cup fresh basil leaves, chopped
- 2 cloves garlic, minced
- 2 tablespoons olive oil
- Salt and pepper to taste

Instructions:

1. Preheat the oven to 375°F (190°C).

2. Cut the spaghetti squash in half lengthwise and scoop out the seeds.

3. Place the squash halves, cut side down, on a baking sheet.

4. Bake for 35-45 minutes, or until the squash is tender and the strands can be easily scraped with a fork.

5. While the squash is baking, prepare the tomato basil sauce by heating olive oil in a skillet over medium heat.

6. Add minced garlic and sauté for 1 minute.

7. Stir in diced tomatoes, fresh basil, salt, and pepper. Simmer for 10-15 minutes.

8. Once the squash is ready, scrape the flesh with a fork to create "spaghetti" strands.

9. Serve the squash with tomato basil sauce on top.

Cooking Time: 50 minutes (including squash baking time).

7. Baked Sweet Potato with Chickpea and Spinach Topping

Baked sweet potatoes topped with chickpeas and spinach are a wholesome and nutrient-dense dinner option that provides fiber and essential nutrients.

Ingredients:

- 2 large sweet potatoes
- 1 can (15 oz) chickpeas, rinsed and drained
- 2 cups fresh spinach
- 1/2 teaspoon cumin

- 1/2 teaspoon paprika

- Salt and pepper to taste

- Olive oil for drizzling

Instructions:

1. Preheat the oven to 400°F (200°C).

2. Wash and scrub the sweet potatoes, then prick them with a fork.

3. Place the sweet potatoes on a baking sheet and bake for 40-50 minutes, or until tender.

4. While the sweet potatoes are baking, heat olive oil in a skillet over medium heat.

5. Add chickpeas, cumin, paprika, salt, and pepper. Sauté for 5 minutes.

6. Stir in fresh spinach and cook until wilted.

7. Once the sweet potatoes are done, cut them open and fluff the flesh with a fork.

8. Top with the chickpea and spinach mixture.

9. Serve hot.

Cooking Time: 60 minutes (including sweet potato baking time).

8. Beef and Vegetable Stir-Fry

A beef and vegetable stir-fry is a protein-packed dinner option filled with colorful veggies, perfect for a balanced menopause diet.

Ingredients:

- 1 pound lean beef (sirloin or flank steak), thinly sliced
- 2 cups mixed vegetables (bell peppers, broccoli, snap peas, carrots)
- 2 cloves garlic, minced
- 1/4 cup low-sodium soy sauce
- 1 tablespoon olive oil
- 1 tablespoon cornstarch (optional, for thickening)
- Cooked brown rice for serving

Instructions:

1. In a bowl, mix soy sauce and cornstarch (if using).

2. Heat olive oil in a skillet or wok over high heat.

3. Add sliced beef and stir-fry for 2-3 minutes until browned. Remove from the skillet and set aside.

4. In the same skillet, add minced garlic and mixed vegetables. Stir-fry until vegetables are tender-crisp.

5. Return the cooked beef to the skillet and pour the soy sauce mixture over it.

6. Stir-fry for an additional 2 minutes, until the sauce thickens.

7. Serve over cooked brown rice.

Cooking Time: 25 minutes.

9. Tofu and Vegetable Curry

A tofu and vegetable curry is a flavorful and vegetarian dinner option rich in protein and fiber, perfect for supporting your menopause diet.

Ingredients:

- 1 block firm tofu, cubed
- 2 cups mixed vegetables (bell peppers, broccoli, carrots), sliced
- 1 onion, finely chopped
- 2 cloves garlic, minced
- 1-inch piece of ginger, minced
- 1 can (14 oz) diced tomatoes
- 2 teaspoons curry powder
- 1 teaspoon cumin

- 1 teaspoon coriander
- Salt and pepper to taste
- Olive oil for cooking
- Fresh cilantro for garnish

Instructions:

1. Heat olive oil in a large skillet over medium heat.

2. Add chopped onion and sauté until translucent.

3. Stir in minced garlic and ginger and cook for another minute.

4. Add diced tomatoes, cubed tofu, curry powder, cumin, coriander, salt, and pepper.

5. Simmer for 20-25 minutes, or until tofu is heated through, stirring occasionally.

6. Just before serving, add mixed vegetables and cook until they are tender-crisp.

7. Garnish with fresh cilantro.

8. Serve with rice or whole-grain bread.

Cooking Time: 45 minutes.

10. Baked Cod with Lemon and Herbs

Baked cod with lemon and herbs is a light and protein-rich dinner option that's easy to prepare.

Ingredients:

- 4 cod fillets
- Zest and juice of 1 lemon
- 2 tablespoons fresh herbs (dill, parsley, thyme), chopped
- 2 cloves garlic, minced
- Olive oil for drizzling
- Salt and pepper to taste

Instructions:

1. Preheat the oven to 375°F (190°C).

2. Place cod fillets on a baking sheet.

3. In a bowl, mix lemon zest, lemon juice, chopped herbs, minced garlic, salt, and pepper.

4. Drizzle the mixture over the cod.

5. Drizzle with olive oil.

6. Bake for 15-20 minutes, or until the cod flakes easily.

7. Serve hot.

Cooking Time: 20 minutes.

Menopause Diet Snack Recipes

1. Greek Yogurt with Berries

Greek yogurt with berries is a quick and nutritious snack that provides calcium and antioxidants to support bone health and combat menopausal symptoms.

Ingredients:

-   1/2 cup Greek yogurt
-   1/4 cup mixed berries (blueberries, strawberries, raspberries)
-   1 teaspoon honey (optional)

Instructions:

1. In a bowl, spoon Greek yogurt.

2. Top with mixed berries.

3. Drizzle with honey if desired.

4. Enjoy!

Preparation Time: 5 minutes.

2. Nut Butter and Banana

Nut butter and banana slices provide healthy fats and potassium, which can help alleviate menopause-related mood swings and muscle cramps.

Ingredients:

- 1 medium ripe banana
- 2 tablespoons almond or peanut butter

Instructions:

1. Slice the banana into rounds.

2. Spread almond or peanut butter on each banana slice.

3. Arrange on a plate or tray.

4. Snack away!

Preparation Time: 3 minutes.

3. Veggie Sticks with Hummus

Fresh veggie sticks paired with hummus make for a crunchy and satisfying snack loaded with fiber and essential nutrients.

Ingredients:

- Carrot sticks
- Celery sticks
- Cucumber slices
- Cherry tomatoes
- Hummus for dipping

Instructions:

1. Wash and chop the vegetables into sticks and slices.

2. Arrange them on a plate with a side of hummus.

3. Dip and enjoy!

Preparation Time: 10 minutes.

4. Trail Mix

A homemade trail mix is a customizable and energy-boosting snack that combines nuts, seeds, and dried fruits for a healthy dose of nutrients.

Ingredients:

- 1/4 cup almonds
- 1/4 cup walnuts
- 1/4 cup pumpkin seeds
- 1/4 cup dried cranberries
- 1/4 cup dark chocolate chips (optional)

Instructions:

1. Mix all the ingredients in a bowl.

2. Portion into snack-sized bags for easy, on-the-go access.

3. Enjoy as needed!

Preparation Time: 5 minutes.

5. Cottage Cheese with Pineapple

Cottage cheese with pineapple chunks is a high-protein snack that provides calcium and vitamin C, which can support bone health and boost the immune system.

Ingredients:

- 1/2 cup low-fat cottage cheese
- 1/4 cup fresh pineapple chunks

Instructions:

1. Spoon cottage cheese into a bowl.

2. Top with pineapple chunks.

3. Dive in!

Preparation Time: 3 minutes.

6. Cucumber Avocado Bites

Cucumber avocado bites are a refreshing and nutrient-rich snack that offers healthy fats and hydration.

Ingredients:

- 1 cucumber, sliced into rounds
- 1/2 avocado, sliced
- Cherry tomatoes, halved
- Fresh basil leaves
- Olive oil drizzle (optional)
- Balsamic glaze drizzle (optional)

Instructions:

1. Place cucumber rounds on a plate.

2. Top each cucumber round with avocado, cherry tomato half, and a fresh basil leaf.

3. Drizzle with olive oil and balsamic glaze if desired.

4. Enjoy the cool, crisp bites!

Preparation Time: 10 minutes.

7. Roasted Chickpeas

Roasted chickpeas are a crunchy, protein-packed snack that provides fiber and essential nutrients to support your menopause diet.

Ingredients:

- 1 can (15 oz) chickpeas, rinsed and drained
- 1 tablespoon olive oil
- 1 teaspoon paprika
- 1/2 teaspoon cumin
- Salt and pepper to taste

Instructions:

1. Preheat the oven to 400°F (200°C).

2. In a bowl, toss chickpeas with olive oil, paprika, cumin, salt, and pepper.

3. Spread the chickpeas on a baking sheet in a single layer.

4. Bake for 25-30 minutes, stirring occasionally until they are crispy.

5. Allow them to cool before snacking.

Preparation Time: 35 minutes.

8. Apple Slices with Almond Butter

Apple slices paired with almond butter provide a satisfying combination of fiber, healthy fats, and vitamins.

Ingredients:

- 1 apple, sliced
- 2 tablespoons almond butter

Instructions:

1. Slice the apple into rounds.

2. Spread almond butter on each apple slice.

3. Arrange on a plate.

4. Enjoy this sweet and nutty snack!

Preparation Time: 5 minutes.

9. Edamame

Edamame (young soybeans) is a protein-rich and low-calorie snack that provides essential nutrients to support your menopause diet.

Ingredients:

- 1 cup frozen edamame pods
- Salt for seasoning (optional)

Instructions:

1. Boil edamame pods in salted water for 3-5 minutes or until tender.

2. Drain and rinse with cold water.

3. Sprinkle with salt if desired.

4. Enjoy these tasty and nutritious beans!

Preparation Time: 10 minutes.

10. Whole Grain Crackers with Tuna Salad

Whole grain crackers with tuna salad make for a protein-packed and satisfying snack, perfect for keeping your energy up during the day.

Ingredients:

- Whole grain crackers
- 1 can (5 oz) tuna, drained
- 2 tablespoons Greek yogurt
- 1 tablespoon chopped celery
- 1 tablespoon diced red onion
- 1 teaspoon Dijon mustard
- Salt and pepper to taste

Instructions:

1. In a bowl, mix tuna, Greek yogurt, celery, red onion, Dijon mustard, salt, and pepper.

2. Spoon the tuna salad onto whole grain crackers.

3. Enjoy this crunchy and creamy snack!

Preparation Time: 10 minutes.

CONCLUSION

In conclusion, a well-balanced menopause diet plays a pivotal role in helping women navigate the physical and emotional changes that come with this life stage. Menopause is a natural transition, and while it may bring challenges, it also presents an opportunity to prioritize health and well-being through dietary choices.

A key focus of the menopause diet is to alleviate the common symptoms of this phase, such as hot flashes, mood swings, and weight gain.

This can be achieved by incorporating foods rich in nutrients like calcium, vitamin D, and omega-3 fatty acids. Calcium and vitamin D support bone health, helping to reduce the risk of osteoporosis, while omega-3 fatty acids can help manage mood swings and inflammation.

Furthermore, maintaining a healthy weight is crucial during menopause, as it can help manage hormonal fluctuations and reduce the risk of chronic diseases. A diet rich in fiber, lean proteins, whole grains, and plenty of fruits and vegetables can aid in weight management and support overall health.

It's important to note that every woman's experience with menopause is unique, and dietary needs may vary. Consulting with a healthcare provider or a registered dietitian is recommended to create a personalized menopause diet plan tailored to individual needs and preferences.

In addition to specific foods, hydration is vital during menopause. Drinking enough water can help alleviate symptoms like hot flashes and promote healthy digestion.

Overall, the menopause diet should emphasize whole, nutrient-dense foods while limiting processed and sugary items. Regular exercise, stress management, and adequate sleep also play important roles in managing menopausal symptoms and overall health.

By embracing a menopause diet that includes a variety of nutrient-rich foods, women can not only ease the transition through this phase but also support their long-term health and well-being. With the right approach to nutrition and lifestyle, menopause can be a time of positive change and renewed vitality.